A
Recommendation
of
Inoculation

According to
Baron Dimsdale's Method

with a facsimile of the original

John Morgan, M.D., F.R.S.

Edited by Matthew T. Colo

NOTE

This recommendation was intended as a preface for the American edition of Baron Thomas Dimsdale's *The present method of inoculating for the smallpox*. However, the edition was never published leading to a separate release of *A Recommendation of Inoculation* with the advertisement included.

ADVERTISEMENT

As it is not unlikely the Smallpox may spread in this Country, it has been thought that the republication of Dimsdale's method of inoculation might be very reasonable at this time, and not less useful. In case the practice of inoculation should hereafter be permitted, the writer of the following pages was requested to favor the editor with a recommendatory preface, to which he readily consented, not doubting its being received with candor; as a desire of being serviceable to the community, was the motive for complying with that request. Being written in haste, and amidst a hurry of business, the indulgent reader will, it is presumed, kindly overlook any inaccuracies that have arisen from his not having had it in his power to devote but a few hours to this otherwise agreeable task.

RECOMMENDATORY PREFACE

It is the opinion of some very observant men that there are few persons but what have the Smallpox at some period of their lives. According to them, at least a fourteenth part of all that are born into the world, die of it. Of those who get it in the natural way, on the most moderate estimation, if we can trust to the reflections of Monsieur Gattie, (to whom the world is indebted for his many other useful remarks on the subject;) the proportion that dies, to those that recover, is as one to ten.[1] Certain it is that a great number of the human race are swept away by its fatal influences; for ever since it has made its first appearance in the known parts of the world, it has marked its course, by the terror, death and devastation that have attended its progress; and has taken off more of the human race than war itself. Next to luxury, ambition and the pride of kings, this appears to be the severest scourge that ever afflicted the unhappy race of man. Villages, towns and cities have been frequently laid waste by it; and entire communities thinned of their inhabitants.

As there is no disease so universal, and at the same time so mortal, there is none which has afforded more exercise to the fancy of speculative men; none concerning which they have entertained a greater variety of opinions, or more false and destructive errors than this. Milled by vain and imaginary hypotheses, they have often rendered this disease,

---

[1] D'après les Calculs les plus modérés la quatorzieme partie des hommes naissent meurent de la petite, vérole, & sur ceux qui sont attaqués de cette cruelle maladie, le nombre de ceux qui en meurent, est au nombre de ceux qui en réchappent, selon quelques ecrivains, comme un à dix; selon d'autres, comme un à sept; et en particulier, d'après celles que l'Hôpital de l'inoculation de Londres vient de fournir, comme un à quatre.—

Gatti, Angelo. *Réfléxions sur les Préjugés qui s'opposent aux progrès et a la perfection de l'inoculation.* p. 88.

so noxious in itself, still more fatal. By the heating method they employed in the management of it, they added fuel to the flame, and armed the disease with a tenfold violence. Long did this mischievous treatment prevail, till our celebrated countryman arose, who may be deservedly styled the British Hippocrates; I mean Sydenham of immortal name. At the head of those few who chose nature for their guide, he opposed the ruinous torrent. Blessed with an uncommon elevation of genius and solid judgment, by a strict attention to facts and useful observations, he laid the foundation of a better and more successful practice. To him we are chiefly beholden for the introduction of a cool regimen in the treatment of the smallpox; and though it did not immediately and extensively prevail, (so great is the power of even the most fatal habits, rooted prejudices and the authority of great names;) yet in after times, when the force of them were dispelled, the minds of men being cleared from the mist, which at first obscured them, became open to conviction, and, at this day, from the difference of treatment, few traces are left of the former mortal effects of the disease. Unspeakable are our obligations, therefore, to this great man, whose history and exact description of the symptoms of the natural smallpox with his method of cure, being founded on the immutable laws of nature, will endure thro' the lapse of time, bid defiance to the cavils of skepticism, and mock the weak attempts of impotent critics to injure or overturn it. The renowned Boerhaave, venerable for his great erudition and profound knowledge of the healing arts, after a laborious perusal of everything written, in his time, on the subject, declares "there is nothing to be added to what Sydenham has delivered on the natural smallpox."

Notwithstanding all the advantages which we derive from the greatest skill in its treatment, it, nevertheless, is at all times, one of the most dangerous diseases that infests the body, when taken in the natural way. In the various expedients that have been devised to mitigate the severity of morbid affections, and to render those which are dangerous, mild and innocent, no invention, surely, (if it may be called an invention, and not rather the inspiration of Heaven itself in pity to man) no attempt to disarm a fatal disease of its violence, was ever so successful, or ever equal in its importance, to that of inoculation properly managed.

When we consider, therefore, the direful effects which commonly attend the natural smallpox, compared with the mildness of its symptoms, and the little danger that accompanies the same disorder by inoculation, we are not surprised that the practice of this art, in spite of every contrivance that has been employed to discredit it, at different times, by a variety of interested men, should triumph at length over all opposition and over the fears and prejudices of weak minded persons, and at this day be so extensively exercised. We have room rather to wonder that it is not universal, or that there is a single person to be met with, who can think of opposing, or neglecting to call in its aid to himself and family, when the disorder appears, and whilst the means of inoculation are within his power.

It is speaking with the greatest caution, simply to affirm, "that the small pox by inoculation, is always much lighter than the natural; that it is a far less dangerous disorder, and is generally benign whenever the subject is well chosen." So great, too, are the improvements that have been made of late years in the practice of inoculation, the preparation of the subject, and treatment of the disease, that it is rare for a patient to be confined one day by it, and we seldom meet with any of those troublesome symptoms that used sometimes to ensue in the neighborhood of the incision, for want of a better method of performing the operation, owing to a groundless apprehension which prevailed, that in any other way, the disorder would not take. There are but few now conversant in the practice, who will allow that those who die from inoculation exceed one in a thousand of those who take the small pox that way; and we hear of some who have inoculated several thousands, successfully, without a single miscarriage. Can there be a stronger argument than this, in favor of the operation, especially when we further add, that wherever it has been practiced, even by the most illiterate persons, it has always been attended with remarkable success?

Not to take up too much time on a subject that has given employment to so many able pens, I shall satisfy myself, for the present, in just pointing at a few of the advantages arising from this practice. And those such as are obvious to everyone who will allow himself to reflect ever so little upon its salutary effects. In the first place then, it is highly beneficial to the patient, that he has it in his power to receive the disease from a healthy subject, in its mildest state, and in the safest manner, and in the absence of every other disease. The choice of the patient's age, of the temperature of the air, season of the year, states of the blood, and general habit of the body, "*free from gouty, rheumatic, scorbutic, inflammatory, or feverish dispositions of every kind,*" as well as of every acute or critical disease with their effects, which render those who labor under them more unfit subjects of inoculation, are none of the most inconsiderable benefits which may be derived from the taking the disease in this way. Yet those are not all; there is some advantage in a suitable preparation of the person to receive the smallpox, from procuring the circumstances necessary for having it with the least possible inconveniency or danger.

I would not here be understood to mean that every person to be inoculated, ought to go through a course of medicine; or that any particular rule can be laid down that will apply precisely to every case. Whilst "those who are in high health or of a plethoric habit of body, require to be reduced to a more secure state; those who are weak and low to be recruited, and those who about with crudities, or sharp humors, to have them corrected or expelled"; so there are some persons who need no preparation whatever; and in whom no change can be made in their constitution, whether by diet or medicine, that will not, by removing it from that exact medium of disposition, in which the most perfect state of health consists, prove hurtful rather than serviceable, and dispose them to have the disease more unfavorably, than if they were to be inoculated without using any medical assistance at all; but these cases are perhaps few: And such persons, when no ways prepared, have from inoculation alone, and a care to avoid all errors in the non-naturals, had the smallpox in the slightest degree, and most favorable manner possible.

The conditions necessary for this purpose, whether natural or acquired by preparation, are "healthy subjects, a sweet breath, a soft skin, and such a disposition of the juices, that a slight wound or scarification with speedily heal."[2] These denote a healthy state of the blood as well as of the nerves and skin, on which the effects of the disease very much depends, and although those conditions tend greatly to render the disease mild, whether taken in the natural way, or by inoculation, yet independently of every other circumstance, it may be said very truly in praise of inoculation, that it contributes greatly to render the disease more mild and safe in itself.

Of this we need no greater proof than what Mr. Gatti produces;[3] he asserts that in the Levant where the smallpox, taken in the natural way, is always as mortal as in other places, inoculation is ever void of danger. There we meet with women who have inoculated thousands without any dangerous accident having befallen any of them, and the only preparation they regard is, to see that the subjects of the operation are suitably prepared to their hands by nature, and have the conditions already enumerated; wherefore we have reason to believe that among all the advantages from inoculation, the greatest of all is the power of choosing in what part of the body, the variolous matter shall enter. In

---

[2] Gatti, Angelo. *Réfléxions sur les Préjugés qui s'opposent aux progrès et a la perfection de l'inoculation.* p. 67.

[3] Ibid. p. 67.

the natural smallpox, the contagion is most commonly taken into the stomach, in deglutition, or applied immediately to the brain and lungs by respiration, organs of the most delicate kind, and whose actions are most essential to life; here the variolous matter by exerting its whole undiminished force, acts with all the energy of its poisonous quality, to injure the blood and nerves, and produces the most fatal effects, whilst in the other way, being received in a very small quantity, by a very slight incision in the skin, it must pass through the lymphatic vessels and glands, which serve as strainers, and which do not suffer it to enter the blood, without being first diluted with lymph in its course to them, through the vessels of absorption, which convey the smallest portion of it, mixed with a very great proportion of lymph, and therefore in a vastly weakened state, first to the glands, and from thence to the blood itself.

In respect to the choice of matter for inoculation, the principle circumstance to be attended to, is that it ought to be taken from a patient who has the large distinct kind, before the decline of the disease, and that is free from every contagious disorder.

From these circumstances which incontestably prove the great benefits arising from inoculation, being now well known and established, the practice of it in America is become very general in the middle colonies; from whence, together with the improvements of employing a cooler regimen, a milder preparation, and the smallness of the incision for engrafting the variolous matter, the smallpox is now disarmed of its former terrors, and become an innocent disease. But the devastations which it has formerly made in New England, in the natural way, and the apprehensions which have filled the minds of many, concerning its fatal effects, have made the inhabitants of these northern colonies take great pains to prevent its getting a footing here; by this means it has been kept out from among them, for a great number of years, till within a twelve month past, during which time it has been introduced by the British troops, into the town of Boston; and inoculation, which was formerly common enough, been generally employed again, with the greatest success: In the mean while from the communication betwixt the town and country being cut off, and the pains taken to prevent its spreading through the country, whenever it had made its appearance there, it has been almost wholly confined to the city.

But since the late rendition of Boston to the American arms from the numbers who have had the disease to recent, and those who were left behind with the small pox upon them, and from the infection that may be supposed to remain for a long time in the bedding and houses of those who have had it; as well as from its having broken out among the soldiery, few of whom have ever had the disorder, there is room to imagine notwithstanding all the precaution taken to prevent, that it will now spread through the country, and perhaps from the marching the troops, backwards and forwards, and the continual moving of the inhabitants to and from Boston, it may now become general through all the New England governments.

In so delicate a juncture when we are struggling with an oppressive war, what an addition must it prove to the burden, should the smallpox spread fast in the natural way; and what an advantage must it be to render inoculation familiar every-where, and to have a sufficient number of practitioners at hand, who are experienced in the treatment of the disease, and who are well acquainted with the practice and late improvement of inoculation? Any attempt to render the knowledge of this matter more general, by removing every prejudice against it, or by recommending to public notice the best treatises on the subject by those who have experienced the good effects of the practice they recommend, I think cannot fail of being received with candor. In that view, I now presume to urge the good people of this country to the perusal of the following treatise, on the present method of inoculation, by the illustrious and deservedly celebrated Baron Dimsdale, to whom both Europe and America will be ever indebted for his improvements in inoculation and the treatment of the disease, and who has carried the benefits arising from the effects much farther than was ever practiced by any of his predecessors, not excepting the great Sydenham himself.

His method like that of Sydenham, proceeding on the sure ground of experiment and observation, is founded on plain facts, simple and uniform, in which he appears not to have suffered the illusions of mere theory, to have usurped the place of experience, or to have perverted his judgment. The good effects of his method are confirmed by the united suffrages of the best practitioners, and have established his character on the most solid basis. His talents and great reputation are well known in the literary world. The utility of the work and the favorable reception its first appearance met with from the public, as well as the avidity with which its several editions have been received, may justly supersede every other eulogy, and render any apology for its publication, at this time, unnecessary; nor have I the vanity to imagine my approbation is needed, or can stamp any value on the performance. There are few persons who need be told, that his eminence in his profession, and the success of his practice, in the treatment of the disease, procured his being sent from Great-Britain to the court of Muscovy, to inoculate the Russian

Empress and her Son; that he was ennobled for this service and was made body physician to her Imperial Majesty; and after inoculating many of the first personages in the empire, successfully, he returned home crowned with honors.

If I mistake not the exact epoch, it was just at a time when that magnanimous Princess was about to engage in war with so formidable a power as the Turks, and in which she came off so victorious. Far from dreading the consequence of inoculation, at so critical a period, she judged it to be a matter of the highest importance, to secure against taking the smallpox in the natural way, which the war might otherwise introduce, and the fear of its dreadful effects might impede the operation of her arms. In that particular, she has held forth an example worthy of our imitation, and which by the event proved the wisdom of the measure.

From the present posture of public affairs and the moral impracticability of preventing the spreading of the smallpox in the natural way, nothing can be more interesting to this country, than the manner in which the present attempt to introduce inoculation may be received and encouraged. If it were once to establish itself in this province it would be the surest means of extending its salutary influence throughout the neighboring colonies that are in a similar situation, and the practice of it being kept up, the disorder would never become formidable again, nor excite that panic it has often done in times past.

Happy for mankind, wherever inoculation has once had a fair trial, those prejudices, that are apt to infect vulgar and weak minds, soon vanish, from the advantages that attend the practice of it. Formerly there were some, otherwise, sensible people, so alarmed about the consequence of the operation, as to think *"the smallpox by inoculation as dangerous, as when taken the natural way; and that it was* contrary to morality and religion to practice it." The former of these objections to it, I hope, I have fully anticipated, and shewn them to be destitute of truth; and in answer to the latter, I shall just observe, that in the middle colonies of America, particularly in Pennsylvania, the Jerseys and New-York, where the disease has long been endemial, from the universal practice of inoculation, it has become in a manner harmless, and there are few people to have the disease but infants and strangers. There, instead of considering it as a crime to inoculate, people would accuse themselves of being accessary to the death of such as fell a sacrifice to the natural smallpox, if, by their neglect the operation had been omitted. They take care to have all under their charge inoculated, when at the most suitable age for taking the disease, esteeming themselves responsible to their children and families, whose preservation they are bound to consult; and to the community of which they are members.

It may be there are some humane persons who have no objection against inoculation themselves, who, nevertheless, think "the apprehension of those, who have never had the disease is a sufficient reason for disallowing the practice of it in others." If this be admitted as satisfactory where the disease has not made its appearance, and is in no danger of spreading; "are not the fears of those, on the other hand, of equal force and validity in favor of inoculation, who are exposed to take the infection, least they should be seized with it in the natural way; and is it not equally just that those persons should be allowed to guard themselves and their families from the dangerous effects of the natural smallpox, by employing inoculation as that others should forbid them; or is the interest of that part of the community who wish to preserve themselves from the ravages of a destructive disease by means of it, less to be regarded than of that other part who do not choose to practice it? To forbid it, when thus circumstanced, is a greater violation of the natural rights of mankind to make use of the means of self-preservation, than to employ them, though others may be averse to the measure; especially when the society at large is benefited by it". How wise is it, then, in every community, where there is danger of spreading the disease, to provide for the safety of its members by rendering the practice of inoculation as universal as possible.

By it whole countries are freed from constant dread of the mischiefs that might arise from its racing amongst them, at a time when they are least prepared, and when few amongst them having had the disease, are in a situation to succor their friends, by which means, thousands fall daily victims to its destructive rage.

The subject is important, and the public is greatly interested in it; and not the less so that is has been so comparatively little practiced, and therefore is yet so new to many in this country. In the treatment of diseases, mistakes at first have a fatal tendency, and there is a necessity of a skillful director, to prevent the errors on account of the pernicious consequences of them, which acquire an establishment by time, custom or great authorities. These, I imagine, Dimsdale's treatise will have a happy tendency to prevent, by rendering the practice of inoculation more familiar and better understood. To those who have not had much opportunity of seeing in what manner any physical operation is best managed, or how a particular disease is treated with the greatest success, it will always be of infinite advantage to avail themselves of the assistance of a skillful pilot. Nature conceals many of her works so closely as often to elude the researches of the most inquisitive, and requires the experience of others to point them out.

This author's practice will cast great light on the business of inoculation, and serve as a clue to guide the attentive follower in the treatment of a disease in which the most clear sighted often have occasion of help to shun danger, and to conduct those who are committed to their care through the disorder, with satisfaction and honor to themselves, and benefit to the community. In the account which our author has given us of his practice of inoculation and treatment of the sick, he has laid down ample directions, and all along, expressed himself with remarkable perspicuity, and as much elegance of diction, as the subject will admit.

From the experience I have had of the good effects of Dimsdale's method of inoculation, I imagine, in recommending it to such practitioners as may be shortly engaged in taking care of those, amongst whom the smallpox may spread, and particularly to the surgeons of the hospital, and those in the army under my own direction, I am performing one of the most important services a person in my station can well render to them, or to the country and people he is amongst. Every attempt to spread the knowledge of any useful practice, has a natural tendency to advance science and redound to the public good. All the merit I propose to myself in the recommendation of the author, is the holding him forth to more public view, and a desire to excite a general attention to so valuable a performance amongst some who may be less acquainted with its value. As the public good is my intention in this, I flatter myself I shall attain my wish, being persuaded that no person who shall carefully read the following sheets, and attend to the information they contain will think their time misapplied, or repent their having followed so safe and experienced a guide in the practice of inoculation.

John Morgan

Cambridge, in New England
April 19th 1776.

A

RECOMMENDATION

OF

INOCULATION,

ACCORDING TO

BARON DIMSDALE's METHOD.

BY JOHN MORGAN, MD, FRS, &c.
DIRECTOR-GENERAL OF THE HOSPITALS, AND
PHYSICIAN IN CHIEF OF THE *AMERICAN* ARMY.

BOSTON.

PRINTED BY J. GILL, IN QUEEN-STREET.

M,DCC,LXXVI.

ADVERTISEMENT.

AS it is not unlikely the Small-Pox may spread in this Country, it has been thought that the republication of Dimsdale's *method of inoculation might be very seasonable at this time, and not less useful. In case the practice of inoculation should hereafter be permitted, the writer of the following pages was requested to favour the editor with a recommendatory preface, to which he readily consented, not doubting it's being received with candor ; as a desire of being serviceable to the community, was the motive for complying with that request. Being written in haste, and amidst a hurry of business, the indulgent reader will, it is presumed, kindly overlook any inaccuracies that have arisen from his not having had it in his power to devote but a few hours to this otherwise agreeable task.*

RECOMMENDATORY PREFACE.

IT is the opinion of fome very obfervant men that there are few perfons but what have the Small-Pox at fome period of their lives. According to them, at leaft a fourteenth part of all that are born into the world, die of it. Of thofe who get it in the natural way, on the moft moderate eftimation, if we can truft to the reflections of Monfieur Gatti, (to whom the world is indebted for his many other ufeful remarks on the fubject ;) the proportion that die, to thofe that recover, is as one to ten. * Certain it is that a great number of the human race are fwept away by its fatal influence ; for ever fince it has made its firft appearance in the known parts of the world, it has marked its courfe, by the terror,

A 2

death

* D'apiès les Calculs les plus modérés la quatorzieme partie des hommes naiffent meuient de la petite, verole, & fur ceux qui font attaqués de cette cruelle maladie, le nombre de ceux qui en muient, eft au nombre de ceux qui en rechappent, felon quelques ecrivains, comme un a dix ; felon d'autres, comme un à fept ; et enfin d'aupres quelques tables, et en particulier, d'après celles que l' Hofpital de l' inoculation de Londres vient de fournir, comma un a quatre.——

Gatti, fur les Préjugés qui s'oppofent au progrès et a la perfection de l'inoculation. p. 88.

death and devaftation that have attended its progrefs ; and has taken off more of the human race than war itfelf. Next to luxury, ambition and the pride of kings, this appears to be the fevereft fcourge that ever afflicted the unhappy race of man. Villages, towns and cities have been frequently laid wafte by it ; and entire communities thinned of their inhabitants.

As there is no difeafe fo univerfal, and at the fame time fo mortal, there is none which has afforded more exercife to the fancy of fpeculative men ; none concerning which they have entertain'd a greater variety of opinions, or more falfe and deftructive errors than this. Mifled by vain and imaginary hypothefes, they have often render'd this difeafe, fo noxious in itfelf, ftill more fatal. By the heating method they employed in the management of it, they added fuel to the flame, and armed the difeafe with a tenfold violence. Long did this mifchievous treatment prevail, till our celebrated countryman arofe, who may be defervedly ftiled the Britifh Hippocrates ; I mean Sydenham of immortal name. At the head of thofe few who chofe nature for their guide, he oppofed the ruinous torrent. Bleffed with an uncommon elevation of genius and folid judgment, by a ftrict attention to facts and ufeful obfervations, he laid the foundation of a better and more fuccefsful practice. To him we are chiefly beholden for the introduction of a cool regimen in the treatment of the fmall-pox ; and tho' it did not immediately and extenfively pre-

vail, (fo great is the power of even the moft fatal
habits, rooted prejudices and the authority of
great names ;) yet in after times,when the force
of them were difpelled, the minds of men being
cleared from the mift which at firft obfcured them,
became open to conviction, and, at this day, from
the difference of treatment, few traces are left
of the former mortal effects of the difeafe. Un-
fpeakable are our obligations, therefore, to this
great man, whofe hiftory and exact defcription
of the fymptoms of the natural fmall-pox with
his method of cure, being founded on the immutable laws of nature, will endure thro' the
lapfe of time, bid defiance to the cavils of fcepti-
cifm, and mock the weak attempts of impotent
critics to injure or overturn it. The renowned
Boerhaave, venerable for his great erudition and
profound knowledge of the healing arts, after a
laborious perufal of every thing written, in his
time, on the fubject, declares " there is nothing
" to be added to what Sydenham has delivered
" on the natural fmall-pox."

Notwithftanding all the advantages which we
derive from the greateft fkill in its treatment, it,
neverthelefs, is at all times, one of the moft dangerous difeafes that infelts the body, when taken
in the natural way. In the various expedients
that have been devifed to mitigate the feverity
of morbid affections, and to render thofe which
are dangerous, mild and innocent, no invention,
furely, (if it may be called an invention, and not
rather the infpiration of Heaven itfelf in pity to

man) no attempt to difarm a fatal difeafe of its violence, was ever fo fuccefsful, or ever equal in its importance, to that of inoculation properly managed.

When we confider, therefore, the direful effects which commonly attend the natural fmall-pox, compared with the mildnefs of its fymptoms, and the little danger that accompanies the fame diforder by inoculation, we are not furprized that the practice of this art, in fpight of every contrivance that has been employed to difcredit it, at different times, by a variety of interefted men, fhould triumph at length over all oppofition and over the fears and prejudices of weak minded perfons, and at this day be fo extenfively exerci-fed. We have room rather to wonder that it is not univerfal, or that there is a fingle perfon to be met with, who can think of oppofing, or neglecting to call in its aid to himfelf and family, when the diforder appears, and whilft the means of inoculation are within his power.

It is fpeaking with the greateft caution, fimply to affirm, " *that the fmall pox by inoculation, is always much lighter than the natural ; that it is a far lefs dangerous diforder, and is generally benign whenever the fubject is well chofen.*" So great, too, are the improvements that have been made of late years in the practice of inoculation, the preparation of the fubject, and treatment of the difeafe, that it is rare for a patient to be confin'd one day by it, and we feldom meet with any of thofe

troublefome

troublesome symptoms that used sometimes to ensue in the neighbourhood of the incision, for want of a better method of performing the operation, owing to a groundless apprehension which prevailed, that in any other way, the disorder would not take. There are but few now conversant in the practice, who will allow that those who die from inoculation exceed one in a thousand of those who take the small pox that way ; and we hear of some who have inoculated several thousands, successfully, without a single miscarriage. Can there be a stronger argument than this, in favour of the operation, especially when we further add, that wherever it has been practised, even by the most illiterate persons, it has always been attended with remarkable success ?

Not to take up too much time on a subject that has given employment to so many able pens, I shall satisfy myself, for the present, in just pointing at a few of the advantages arising from this practice. And those such as are obvious to every one who will allow himself to reflect ever so little upon its salutary effects. In the first place then, it is highly beneficial to the patient, that he has it in his power to receive the disease from a healthy subject, in its mildest state, and in the safest manner, and in the absence of every other disease. The choice of the patient's age, of the temperature of the air, season of the year, state of the blood, and general habit of the body, " *free from gouty, rheumatic, scorbutic, inflammatory,* " *or feverish dispositions of every kind,*" as well as of every

every acute or critical difeafe with their effects, which render thofe who labour under them more unfit fubjects of inoculation, are none of the moft inconfiderable benefits which may be derived from the taking the difeafe in this way. Yet thofe are not all; there is fome advantage in a fuitable preparation of the perfon to receive the fmallpox, from procuring the circumftances neceffary for having it with the leaft poffible inconveniency or danger.

I would not here be underftood to mean that every perfon to be inoculated, ought to go thro' a courfe of medicine; or that any particular rule can be laid down that will apply precifely to every cafe. Whilft "thofe who are in high health or of a " plethoric habit of body, require to be reduced to " a more fecure ftate; thofe who are weak and " low to be recruited, and thofe who abound " with crudities, or fharp humours, to have " them corrected or expelled"; fo there are fome perfons who need no preparation whatever; and in whom no change can be made in their conftitution, whether by diet or medicine, that will not, by removing it from that exact medium of difpofition, in which the moft perfect ftate of health confifts, prove hurtful rather than ferviceable, and difpofe them to have the difeafe more unfavorably, than if they were to be inoculated without ufeing any medical affiftance at all; but thefe cafes are perhaps few: And fuch perfons, when no ways prepared, have from inoculation alone, and a care to avoid all errors in the non-
naturals,

naturals, had the fmall-pox in the flighteft degree, and moft favorable manner poffible.

The conditions neceffary for this purpofe, whether natural or acquired by preparation, are
" healthy fubjects, a fweet breath, a foft fkin,
" and fuch a difpofition of the juices, that a
" flight wound or fcarification will fpeedily
" heal." * Thefe denote a healthy ftate of the
blood as well as of the nerves and fkin, on which
the effects of this difeafe very much depends,
and although thofe conditions tend greatly to
render the difeafe mild, whether taken in the natural way, or by inoculation, yet independently
of every other circumftance, it may be faid very
truly in praife of inoculation, that it contributes
greatly to render the difeafe more mild and fafe
in itfelf.

Of this we need no greater proof than what
Mr Gatti produces †; he afferts that in the Levant where the fmall-pox, taken in the natural
way, is always as mortal as in other places, inoculation is ever void of danger. There we meet
with women who have inoculated thoufands,
without any dangerous accident having befallen
any of them, and the only preparation they regard is, to fee that the fubjects of the operation
are fuitably prepared to their hands by nature,
and have the conditions already enumerated ;
wherefore we have reafon to believe that among
all the advantages from inoculation, the greateft

B   of

of all is the power of choosing in what part of the body, the variolous matter shall enter. In the natural small-pox, the contagion is most commonly taken into the stomach, in deglutition, or apply'd immediately to the brain and lungs by respiration, organs of the most delicate kind, and whose actions are most essential to life; here the variolous matter by exerting its whole undiminished force, acts with all the energy of its poisonous quality, to injure the blood and nerves, and produces the most fatal effects, whilst in the other way, being received in a very small quantity, by a very slight incision in the skin, it must pass through the lymphatic vessels and glands, which serve as strainers, and which do not suffer it to enter the blood, without being first diluted with lymph in its course to them, through the vessels of absorption, which convey the smallest portion of it, mixed with a very great proportion of lymph, and therefore in a vastly weakened state, first to the glands, and from thence to the blood itself.

In respect to the choice of matter for inoculation, the principle circumstance to be attended to, is that it ought to be taken from a patient who has the large distinct kind, before the decline of the disease, and that is free from every contagious disorder.

From these circumstances which incontestably prove the great benefits arising from inoculation, being now well known and established, the practice

tice of it in America is become very general in the middle colonies ; from whence, together with the improvements of employing a cooler regimen, a milder preparation, and the fmalinefs of the incifion for ingrafting the variolous matter, the fmall-pox is now difarmed of its former terrors, and become an innocent difeafe. But the devaftations which it has formerly made in New-England, in the natural way, and the apprehenfions which have filled the minds of many, concerning its fatal effects, have made the inhabitants of thefe nothern colonies take great pains to prevent its getting a footing here ; by this means it has been kept out from among them, for a great number of years, till within a twelve month paft, during which time it has been introduced by the Britifh troops, into the town of Bofton ; and inoculation, which was formerly common enough, been generally employed again, with the greateft fuccefs : In the mean while from the communication betwixt the town and country being cut off, and the pains taken to prevent its fpreading through the country, whenever it had made its appearance there, it has been almoft wholly confined to the city.

But fince the late rendition of Bofton to the American arms from the numbers who have had the difeafe fo recent, and thofe who were left behind with the fmall pox upon them, and from the infection that may be fuppofed to remain for a long time in the bedding and houfes of thofe who have had it ; as well as from its having broke

out

out among the foldiery, few of whom have ever had the diforder, there is room to imagine notwithftanding all the precaution taken to prevent, it will now fpread through the country, perhaps from the marching the troops, backwards and forwards, and the continual moving the inhabitants to and from Bofton, it may become general through all the New-England ments.

In fo delicate a juncture when we are ftruggling with an oppreffive war, what an addition muft it prove to the burden, fhould the fmall-pox fpread faft in the natural way ; and what an advantage muft it be to render inoculation familiar every-where, and to have a fufficient number of practitioners at hand, who are experienced in the treatment of the difeafe, and who are well acquainted with the practice and late improvement of inoculation ? Any attempt to render the knowledge of this matter more general, by removing every prejudice againft it, or by recommending to public notice the beft treatifes on the fubject by thofe who have experienced the good effects of the practice they recommend, I think cannot fail of being received with candour. In that view, I now prefume to urge the good people of this country to the perufal of the following treatife, on the prefent method of inoculation, by the illuftrious and defervedly celebrated Baron Dimfdale, to whom both Europe and America will be ever indebted for his improvements in inoculation and the treatment of the difeafe,

and

and who has carry'd the benefits arifing from the effects much farther than was ever practifed by any of his predeceffors, not excepting the great Sydenham himfelf.

His method like that of Sydenham, proceeding on the fure ground of experiment and obfervation, is founded on plain facts, fimple and uniform, in which he appears not to have fuffered the illufions of mere theory, to have ufurped the place of experience, or to have perverted his judgment. The good effects of his method are confirmed by the united fuffrages of the beft practitioners, and have eftablifhed his character on the moft folid bafis. His talents and great reputation are well known in the literary world. The utility of the work and the favourable reception its firft appearance met with from the publick, as well as the avidity with which its feveral editions have been received, may juftly fupercede every other eulogy, and render any apology for its publication, at this time, unneceffary ; nor have I the vanity to imagine my approbation is needed or can ftamp any value on the performance. There are few perfons who need be told, that his eminence in his profeffion, and the fuccefs of his practice, in the treatment of the difeafe, procured his being fent from Great-Britain to the court of Mufcovy, to inoculate the Ruffian Emprefs and her Son ; that he was enobled for this fervice and was made body phyfician to her Imperial Majefty ; and after inoculating many of the firft perfonages in the empire, fuccefsfully, he returned home crowned with honours.

If

If I miftake not the exact epocha, it was juft at a time when that magnanimous Princefs was about to engage in war with fo formidable a power as the Turks, and in which fhe came off fo victorious. Far from dreading the confequence of inoculation, at fo critical a period, fhe judged it to be a matter of the higheft importance, to fecure againft taking the fmall-pox in the natural way, which the war might otherwife introduce, and the fear of its dreadful effects might impede the operation of her arms. In that particular, fhe has held forth an example worthy of our imitation, and which by the event proved the wifdom of the meafure.

From the prefent pofture of public affairs and the moral impracticability of preventing the fpreading of the fmall-pox in the natural way, nothing can be more interefting to this country, than the manner in which the prefent attempt to introduce inoculation may be received and encouraged. If it were once to eftablifh itfelf in this province it would be the fureft means of extending its falutary influence throughout the neighbouring colonies that are in a fimilar fituation, and the practice of it being kept up, the diforder would never become formidable again, nor excite that panick it has often done in times paft.

Happy for mankind, wherever inoculation has once had a fair trial, thofe prejudices, that are apt to infect vulgar and weak minds, foon vanifh, from the advantages that attend the practice of

it. Formerly there were fome, otherwife, fen-
fible people, fo alarmed about the confequence
of the operation, as to think " *the fmall-pox by*
" *inoculation as dangerous, as when taken the natu-*
" *ral way ; and that it was* contrary to morality
" and religion to practife it." The former of thefe
objections to it, I hope, I have fully anticipated,
and fhewn them to be deftitute of truth ; and in
anfwer to the latter, I fhall juft obferve, that in
the middle colonies of America, particularly in
Penfylvania, the Jerfeys and New-York, where
the difeafe has long been endemial, from the u-
niverfal practice of inoculation, it has become in
a manner harmlefs, and there are few people to
have the difeafe but infants and ftrangers. There,
inftead of confidering it as a crime to inoculate,
people would accufe themfelves of being acceffa-
ry to the death of fuch as fell a facrifice to the
natural fmall-pox, if, by their neglect the operation had been omitted. They take care to have
all under their charge inoculated, when at the
moft fuitable age for taking the difeafe, efteeming
themfelves refponfible to their children and families, whofe prefervation they are bound to con-
fult ; and to the community of which they are
members.

It may be there are fome humane perfons who
have no objection againft inoculation themfelves,
who, neverthelefs, think " the apprehenfion of
" thofe, who have never had the difeafe is a fuf-
" ficient reafon for difallowing the practice of it
" in others." If this be admitted as fatisfactory
where

where the difeafe has not made its appearance,
and is in no danger of fpreading ; " are not the
fears of thofe, on the other hand, of equal force
and validity in favour of inoculation, who
are expofed to take the infection, leaft they
fhould be feized with it in the natural way ; and
is it not equally juft that thofe perfons fhould be
allowed to guard themfelves and their families
from the dangerous effects of the natural fmall-
pox, by employing inoculation, as that others
fhould forbid them ; or is the intereft of that
part of the community who wifh to preferve
themfelves from the ravages of a deftructive difeafe by means of it, lefs to be regarded than of
that other part who do not choofe to practife it ?
To forbid it, when thus circumftanced, is a greater volation of the natural rights of mankind to
make ufe of the means of felf-prefervation, than
to employ them, though others may be averfe
to the meafure ; efpecially when the fociety at
large is benefited by it". How wife is it, then,.
in every community, where there is danger of
fpreading the difeafe, to provide for the fafety of
its members by rendering the practice of inoculation as univerfal as poffible.

By it whole countries are freed from conftant
dread of the mifchiefs that might arife from its ra-
ging amongft them, at a time when they are leaft
prepared, and when few amongft them having
had the difeafe, are in a fituation to fuccour their
friends, by which means, thoufands fall daily victims to its deftructive rage.

The

The subject is important, and the publick is greatly interested in it; and not the less so, that it has been so comparatively little practised, and therefore is yet so new to many in this country. In the treatment of diseases, mistakes at first have a fatal tendency, and there is a necessity of a skilful director, to prevent errors on account of the pernicious consequences of them, which acquire an establishment by time, custom or great authorities. These, I imagine, Dimsdale's treatise will have an happy tendency to prevent, by rend'ring the practice of inoculation more familiar and better understood. To those who have not had much opportunity of seeing in what manner any physical operation is best managed, or how a particular disease is treated with the greatest success, it will always be of infinite advantage to avail themselves of the assistance of a skilful pilot. Nature conceals many of her works so closely as often to elude the researches of the most inquisitive, and requires the experience of others to point them out.

This author's practice will cast great light on the business of inoculation, and serve as a clue to guide the attentive follower in the treatment of a disease in which the most clear sighted often have occasion of help to shun danger, and to conduct those who are committed to their care through the disorder, with satisfaction and honour to themselves, and benefit to the community. In the account which our author has given us of his practice of inoculation and treatment
of

of the fick, he has laid down ample directions, and, all along, expreffed himfelf with remarkable perfpicuity, and as much elegance of diction, as the fubject will admit.

From the experience I have had of the good effects of Dimfdale's method of inoculation, I imagine, in recommending it to fuch practitioners as may be fhortly engaged in taking care of thofe, amongft whom the fmall-pox may fpread, and particularly to the furgeons of the hofpital, and thofe in the army under my own direction, I am performing one of the moft important fervices a perfon in my ftation can well render to them, or to the country and people he is amongft. Every attempt to fpread the knowledge of any ufeful practice, has a natural tendency to advance fcience and redound to the publick good. All the merit I propofe to myfelf in the recommendation of this author, is the holding him forth to more publick view, and a defire to excite a general attention to fo valuable a performance amongft fome who may be lefs acquainted with its value. As the publick good is my intention in this, I flatter myfelf I fhall attain my wifh, being perfwaded that no perfon who fhall carefully read the following fheets, and attend to the information they contain will think their time mifapply'd, or repent their having followed fo fafe and experienced a guide in the practice of inoculation.

JOHN MORGAN.

Cambridge, in New-England *April* 19th 1776.

www.ingramcontent.com/pod-product-compliance
Lightning Source LLC
Chambersburg PA
CBHW070926180526
45168CB00005B/2172